ESOPHAGITIS DIET FOR BEGINNERS

Empower Yourself With Nutritional Strategies, Recipes, Meal Plans, And Expert Tips To Alleviate Esophagitis – A Holistic Guide To Eating For Wellness

DR. JACE ZAYDEN

Table of Contents

DISCLAIMER

The information provided in the book is intended for general informational purposes only. The content of this book should not be considered a substitute for professional medical advice, diagnosis, or treatment.

Readers are advised to consult with a qualified healthcare professional for medical advice tailored to their individual circumstances.

The author has made every effort to ensure that the information in this book is accurate and up-to-date at the time of publication. However, medical knowledge is constantly evolving, and new research may emerge that could impact the information presented. The author disclaims any responsibility for any adverse effects or consequences resulting from the use of the information provided in this book.

References or mentions of individuals, products, websites, organizations, or other names within this book are for informational purposes only and do not constitute an endorsement. The author has no affiliations with, and makes no endorsements of, any third-party entities mentioned. Readers are encouraged to conduct their own research and exercise their judgment when considering any external resources or recommendations.

The author and the publisher shall have neither liability nor responsibility to any person or entity with respect to any loss, damage, or injury caused or alleged to be caused directly or indirectly by the information contained in this book. Any reliance on the information within this book is at the reader's own risk.

By reading this book, the reader acknowledges and agrees to the terms of this disclaimer. If the reader does not agree with these terms, they should not use the information provided in this book.

ABOUT THIS BOOK

This book entitled "Esophagitis Diet" functions as an all-encompassing manual for those who are afflicted with esophagitis, a medical condition distinguished by inflammation of the esophagus. The introductory segment offers a fundamental comprehension of esophagitis, thereby setting the stage for the subsequent discourse. About the management of esophagitis, this book provides a comprehensive explanation of how dietary decisions can substantially influence both the severity and advancement of the condition.

The significance of following a customized dietary regimen is emphasized consistently throughout the text. General dietary guidelines function as a foundational structure, furnishing individuals with a comprehensive comprehension of nutritional tenets about the management of esophagitis. This book provides a comprehensive analysis of particular foods that should be incorporated into a diet for esophagitis, offering pragmatic advice on how to construct a meal plan that is both nourishing and soothing. Concurrently, it identifies foods that should be avoided, providing clarification on potential triggers that may worsen symptoms of esophagitis.

The topic of meal planning is thoroughly examined, including the intricacies involved in organizing a diet that promotes alleviation from esophagitis. Practical strategies for managing daily dietary challenges are presented, thereby assisting the reader in coping with esophagitis. The investigation also examines the impact of beverages on esophagitis, providing nuanced suggestions for maintaining adequate hydration and managing symptoms.

Acknowledging the holistic aspect of esophagitis management, this book delves into topics beyond mere dietary factors. Esophagitis symptom relief is commonly attributed to the implementation of lifestyle modifications. A compilation of exemplar esophagitis diet plans accommodates a wide range of preferences, offering readers practical and modifiable resolutions.

Additionally, this book guides cookery and preparation, enabling readers to savor delectable meals while maintaining their esophagitis management objectives intact. It enables readers to acclimate to changing dietary requirements by providing guidance on monitoring and modifying their diets. Constraints regarding the value of seeking guidance from a healthcare professional are consistently emphasized in this book, emphasizing the need for a customized and cooperative strategy to ensure the successful management of esophagitis.

Fundamentally, "Esophagitis Diet" establishes itself as an indispensable resource by merging pragmatic advice with authoritative knowledge to enable users to effectively navigate the intricacies of managing esophagitis using well-informed dietary decisions and modifications to their way of life.

CHAPTER ONE

Introduction

Esophagitis is a pathological state distinguished by inflammation of the esophagus, the antral-gastric conduit. Diverse factors, including gastroesophageal reflux disease (GERD), infections, and specific medications, can contribute to its development. Symptoms frequently encountered by individuals diagnosed with esophagitis include chest pain, difficulty swallowing, and indigestion. A critical component of a holistic approach to esophagitis management is dietary modification. It is critical to develop a suitable Esophagitis Diet to mitigate symptoms and facilitate the recovery process. This article explores multiple facets of the Esophagitis Diet, including the significance of diet in its management and the significance of comprehending the condition. It also provides general dietary recommendations for those who are afflicted with esophagitis.

Comprehension Of Esophagitis

Esophagitis is a pathological state characterized by inflammation and irritation of the esophagus. A prevalent factor is gastroesophageal reflux disease (GERD), which occurs when gastric acid refluxes into the esophagus. Constant acid exposure can cause irritation and harm to the membrane of the esophagus, ultimately culminating in the development of esophagitis.

Infections, medications, and specific medical conditions that compromise the immune system are additional potential causes. Esophagitis may cause indigestion, regurgitation, chest pain, and difficulty swallowing, among other moderate to severe symptoms. Failure to manage chronic esophagitis may result in complications such as esophageal strictures or Barrett's esophagus, a pathological state that elevates the likelihood of developing esophageal cancer.

It is imperative to comprehend the fundamental etiology of esophagitis to implement efficacious treatment. For example, in the case where gastroesophageal reflux disease (GERD) is the principal etiology, remedying acid reflux becomes a critical emphasis in dietary and therapeutic strategies. Lifestyle modifications and the identification of triggers are essential components of esophagitis management, with diet serving as a critical factor in both symptom management and recovery.

Dietary Importance In Esophagitis Management

Dietary decisions are of paramount importance in the management of esophagitis as they facilitate symptom control and foster esophageal lining healing. The primary objective of an Esophagitis Diet is to minimize the risk of acid reflux and reduce irritation. While some foods and beverages may have the potential to worsen symptoms, others may offer solace and facilitate the recovery process.

A key factor in the management of esophagitis is the avoidance of foods that have the potential to induce acid reflux. Acidic foods (e.g., citrus fruits, tomatoes, and their byproducts), in addition to piquant and oily foods, are frequently encountered triggers. Additionally, it is well-known that caffeine and chocolate relax the lower esophageal sphincter, permitting gastric acid to reflux into the esophagus. Mitigating or removing these stimuli can make a substantial contribution to alleviating symptoms.

The inclusion of foods that promote healing and soothe the esophagus is, however, of equal importance. Fruits that do not contain acids, including melons and bananas, are mild on the esophageal membrane. In general, lean proteins, whole cereals, and oats are well-tolerated and supply vital nutrients without exacerbating symptoms.

In addition to meal timing and portion control, additional variables may influence the symptoms of esophagitis. By consuming smaller, more frequent meals as opposed to larger, heavier ones, the risk of acid reflux can be decreased and the stomach from becoming overloaded avoided.

Additionally, it is prudent to refrain from reclining down or retiring to bed immediately following a meal, as doing so may heighten the likelihood of acid regurgitation.

Standard Dietary Recommendations

It is crucial to adhere to a balanced and esophagitis-friendly diet to effectively manage the condition. Consider the following general dietary recommendations:

1. It is advisable to prioritize the inclusion of low-acid foods in one's dietary regimen, including whole cereals, non-citrus fruits, and vegetables. These foods may be gentler on the esophagus and are less likely to induce acid reflux.

2. Lean protein sources, such as poultry, fish, and tofu, should be prioritized. These proteins increase the likelihood that the stomach will not produce acid, thereby facilitating digestion.

3. Prevent Trigger Foods: Recognize and reduce in quantity or eliminate foods that elicit acid reflux. Acidic vegetables, tomatoes, piquant foods,

chocolate, and caffeine are all examples. Maintaining a food journal could be beneficial in monitoring specific triggers.

4. Small, Frequent Meals: Opt for consuming three substantial meals during the day, opt to consume smaller, more frequent meals. Implementing this strategy may aid in the prevention of excessive gastric distention and decrease the probability of acid reflux.

5. Maintaining sufficient hydration with water is essential. Carbonated and acidic beverages should be avoided, as they may irritate the esophagus.

6. Establish a minimum interval of two to three hours between your final meal and slumber. This provides sufficient time for the stomach to cleanse, thereby decreasing the likelihood of acid reflux occurring during the night.

7. If experiencing symptoms during the night, it is advisable to contemplate raising the head of the bed by an approximate distance of 6 to 8 inches.

This can assist gravity in preventing the reflux of gastric acid into the esophagus during sleep.

8. Gradual Alterations: Implement dietary modifications incrementally to provide the body with an opportunity to adapt. Occasionally, abrupt transitions may result in discomfort or digestive complications.

In summary, the management of esophagitis necessitates a comprehensive strategy, with an essential element being an Esophagitis Diet. To alleviate symptoms and facilitate recuperation, it is imperative to incorporate a diet that supports esophageal health, comprehend the condition, and identify triggers.

To guarantee the most effective management of esophagitis and to tailor dietary recommendations to individual requirements, it is recommended to seek guidance from a registered dietitian or a healthcare professional.

Elimination Of Esophagitis Symptoms Via Strategic Nutrition

Esophagitis, which is distinguished by inflammation of the esophagus, is frequently a distressing condition that necessitates modifications to one's way of life, such as dietary modifications. A diet that is sensitive to esophagitis is vital for symptom management and recuperation. This article explores three fundamental components of a diet for esophagitis: recommended foods, prohibited foods, and techniques for meal planning.

CHAPTER TWO

Esophagitis Dietary Components: Nourishment For Recovery

1. The inclusion of non-acidic fruits and vegetables in the diet is crucial for those who have been diagnosed with esophagitis. Bananas, melons, carrots, and spinach are all viable choices that offer vital vitamins and minerals while avoiding exacerbation of inflammation in the esophagus. These dietary items promote holistic health and facilitate the recovery process.

2. Lean protein sources, including poultry, fish, and tofu, are essential constituents of a diet that is conducive to esophagitis. These proteins have a reduced propensity to induce irritation and are simpler to digest. To reduce the likelihood of inducing symptoms, care must be taken to ensure that no added spices or excessive oils are used in their preparation.

3. Complex carbohydrates, such as those found in whole cereals and oats, offer a prolonged supply

of energy while preventing the occurrence of acid reflux. The high fiber content of these foods reduces the likelihood of esophageal irritation and promotes digestive health.

4. Although it is recommended to limit fat consumption, incorporating healthful lipids into one's diet in moderation, such as avocados and olive oil, can have positive effects. These lipids support digestive health and contribute to a balanced diet.

5. Individuals with a healthy tolerance to dairy products may benefit from selecting low-fat or fat-free alternatives, which are rich in protein and calcium. Nevertheless, it is imperative to closely observe individual tolerance levels, as certain individuals with esophagitis may require dairy restriction or avoidance.

6. Herbs and Mild Spices: Although fiery foods are generally not recommended, specific herbs and mild spices can be utilized to enhance flavor without worsening symptoms. Included among

these are ginger, basil, and oregano. By conducting experiments with these, one can improve the gustatory experience of meals while maintaining digestive comfort.

7. Soft and moist foods have the potential to facilitate digestion and mitigate the likelihood of irritation. Soups, stews, and properly prepared grains have the potential to alleviate discomfort in the esophagus while still providing nourishment.

Avoid Foods Listed In The Esophagitis Diet: Avoiding Triggers

1. Acidic Foods and Beverages: To alleviate the symptoms of esophagitis, acidic foods and beverages should be avoided, including citrus fruits, tomatoes, and citrus juices. Additionally, carbonated beverages, coffee, and tea are frequent offenders that should be substituted with non-acidic alternatives.

2. Spicy and peppery foods: In a diet for esophagitis, spices such as chile, pepper, and spicy sauces should be avoided or reduced in quantity because they can be irritating to the

esophagus. By opting for milder substitutes or conducting experiments with botanicals to impart flavor, one can preserve variety while upholding comfort.

3. Foods High in Fat: Frozen foods, fatty meats, and full-fat dairy products are examples of high-fat foods that can relax the lower esophageal sphincter, resulting in increased acid reflux. It is essential to avoid these alternatives to effectively manage symptoms and induce healing.

4. Chocolate and mint have been identified as potential catalysts for esophagitis symptoms due to their ability to relax the esophageal sphincter. A reduction or elimination of chocolate-based and mint-flavored products may aid in the management of symptoms.

5. Caffeine and Alcohol: Both caffeine and alcohol have the potential to aggravate acid reflux and irritation of the esophagus. Consuming caffeinated and alcoholic beverages, such as tea and cola, in moderation or entirely abstained

from, can assist in the efficient management of symptoms.

6. Spicy and processed foods: Due to their high preservative and additive content, processed foods can be difficult on the digestive system. For improved digestive health, spicy munchies and prepackaged meals should be substituted with whole, unprocessed alternatives.

Planning Esophagitis Meals: Achieving A Balance Between Comfort And Nutrition

1. Consistent Small Meals: Individuals diagnosed with esophagitis frequently experience alleviation from symptoms by adhering to a schedule of smaller, more frequent meals spread out throughout the day, as opposed to ingesting three substantial meals. This methodology aids in mitigating the consequences of gastric excess and reduces the likelihood of acid reflux.

2. Chew Thoroughly: Individuals diagnosed with esophagitis must practice proper digestion. By reducing the strain on the esophagus, thorough

chewing aids digestion and reduces the likelihood of irritation.

3. Eating mindfully and methodically enables people to identify their satiety signals, which prevents excess and improves digestion. Reducing distractions during meals can improve concentration on the activity of dining.

4. Adherence to an upright posture during dining can effectively mitigate the retrograde movement of gastric acid into the esophagus. After meals, spending at least 30 minutes seated upright can substantially reduce the risk of acid reflux.

5. Maintaining proper hydration is of the utmost importance; however, it is recommended to consume water between meals as opposed to during them. Overconsumption of fluids during meals has the potential to elevate gastric pressure, which may result in the development of acid reflux.

As a result, adherence to a well-planned meal regimen and judicious selection of foods to incorporate and exclude are essential components of an esophagitis diet. Individual tolerance levels must guide dietary selections to effectively manage symptoms and promote the healing of an inflamed esophagus.

By incorporating these dietary strategies into their routine, in collaboration with medical advice, individuals afflicted with esophagitis can enhance their quality of life and achieve greater comfort and nourishment.

CHAPTER THREE

Guidelines For Eating While Having Esophagitis

Inflammation of the esophagus, the conduit connecting the stomach and pharynx, is referred to as esophagitis. This condition is frequently accompanied by discomfort and pain, which necessitates dietary adjustments to mitigate symptoms and facilitate the recovery process. A suitable diet for esophagitis can be of critical importance in the management of the condition. The following are some dietary recommendations for those with esophagitis.

1. Select Soft, Easy-to-ingest Foods: To reduce the risk of esophageal irritation, choose foods that are soft and easy to ingest. Esophageal health benefits include the consumption of cooked vegetables, well-prepared cereals, and lean protein sources such as poultry or fish. Rough or gritty textures should be avoided, as they may worsen inflammation.

2. Small, Regular Meals: Opt for imbibing substantial meals and instead incorporate smaller, more frequent meals into your daily routine. This reduces the likelihood of stomach acid refluxing into the esophagus by minimizing the pressure on the lower esophageal sphincter and preventing stomach excess.

3. Mindful Chewing: Chew your food thoroughly by taking your time. This facilitates the process of digestion and may decrease the probability of undigested food inducing esophageal irritation. Air may be swallowed during haste or rapid dining, which may exacerbate symptoms.

4. AVOID Trigger Foods: Determine the foods that cause esophagitis symptoms to worsen and eliminate them from your diet. Spicy foods, acidic fruits, tomatoes, chocolate, caffeine, and oily or fried foods are typical triggers. Maintaining a food diary enables you to monitor your meals and discern recurring patterns of discomfort, thereby facilitating the identification of particular triggers that warrant avoidance.

5. It is imperative to be mindful of the timing of your meals. By consuming food too close to slumber, the risk of acid reflux can be increased. By allowing a minimum of two to three hours to pass between your last meal and slumber, you can ensure adequate emptying of your stomach and minimize the risk of experiencing regurgitation during the night.

6. It is essential to maintain an upright posture during and for a minimum of 45 minutes following meals. This can aid in the prevention of reflux of gastric acid into the esophagus. Promptly reclining or lying down following a meal should be avoided, as it may exacerbate acid reflux.

7. Maintain adequate hydration with water; however, restrict sipping to portioned portions during meals. Water can prevent dehydration while maintaining proper digestion by not neutralizing gastric acid, which is vital for bodily function.

8. It is advisable to seek guidance from a healthcare professional before integrating dietary supplements into your regimen, as they may significantly facilitate the healing process. Antioxidants such as zinc, vitamin C, and zinc, which are involved in immune function and tissue repair, may be among these.

9. Non-Citrus Fruits: Apples, avocados, and melons are examples of non-citrus fruits that may be more tolerable than acidic fruits. These fruits are a beneficial addition to a diet that is favorable to esophagitis because they contain vital nutrients.

10. Dietitian Consultation: It is advisable to consult with a registered dietitian for personalized dietary recommendations that address individual requirements. A dictitian can assist in the development of a nutritious and well-balanced meal plan that promotes recovery and reduces discomfort.

Dietary modification for the treatment of esophagitis necessitates deliberate selections that reduce irritation and promote healing. By applying these suggestions, one can potentially alleviate symptoms and improve their general state of health.

The Relationship Between Beverages And Esophagitis

Particularly when managing esophagitis, it is critical to be mindful of beverage selections, as specific beverages have the potential to either worsen or mitigate symptoms. Consuming appropriate beverages can facilitate the healing process and provide relief from esophagitis. The following is a guide to making informed decisions regarding esophagitis and beverages.

1. Water is the most effective beverage for maintaining hydration. It aids in gastric acid diluting and can provide esophageal relief.

To avoid gastric overfilling, consume water in moderation throughout the day, avoiding large portions during meals.

2. Herbal Teas: Herbal teas, including ginger tea and chamomile, may have digestive system-soothing properties. These alternatives devoid of caffeine may assist in mitigating the symptoms associated with esophagitis. It is important to use tepid tea, as heated beverages have the potential to irritate the esophagus.

3. Aloe vera juice, renowned for its anti-inflammatory properties, might offer solace to the symptoms associated with esophagitis. Nevertheless, it is imperative to seek the advice of a healthcare professional before integrating aloe vera into your daily regimen, as its suitability may vary among individuals.

4. Individuals with esophagitis may find coconut water to be a hydrating and low-acid beverage to be tolerable. As an alternative to acidic fruit beverages, it may be invigorating.

5. Although milk is commonly perceived as a calming beverage, it is critical to select low-fat or fat-free alternatives, as the consumption of high-

fat dairy products may elicit acid reflux. A modest serving of chilled milk may provide some individuals with symptomatic alleviation.

6. When considering dietary beverages, it is advisable to choose non-acidic varieties like cabbage or carrot juice to consume vital nutrients without irritating the esophagus. Water should be used to dilute liquids to reduce their acidity.

7. Acidic juices, including tomato juice and citrus juice, should be avoided because they can aggravate the symptoms of esophagitis. Avoid consuming these beverages to protect the already inflamed esophagus from irritation.

8. Limit or eliminate your intake of caffeinated beverages and alcohol, as they have the potential to relax the lower esophageal sphincter and facilitate acid reflux. As alternatives, select decaffeinated coffee and medicinal beverages.

9. Carbonated Beverages: Sodas and other carbonated beverages can increase pressure on the lower esophageal sphincter and contribute to

obesity. Reduce your risk of acid reflux by consuming still water or non-carbonated beverages.

10. Ice Chips: In cases where distress associated with esophagitis hinders the ability to swallow, the analgesic effect of ice chips on the pharynx may offer some solace. However, avoid beverages that are excessively heated or cold, as they may irritate.

To manage esophagitis, it is necessary to modify one's beverage selection to exclude acidic, effervescent, and trigger-inducing beverages while integrating calming alternatives.

Adequate hydration with appropriate beverages can supplement dietary adjustments and aid in the management of esophagitis as a whole.

CHAPTER FOUR

Alterations To One's Lifestyle
Regarding The Esophagitis Diet

Alterations to one's lifestyle, in conjunction with dietary modifications, can substantially contribute to the alleviation of esophagitis. The objective of these alterations is to reduce elements that contribute to inflammation and enhance digestive health as a whole. Key lifestyle modifications to contemplate for the management of esophagitis are as follows.

1. It is imperative to maintain a healthy weight, as surplus weight, particularly in the abdominal region, can exacerbate gastric pressure and potentially exacerbate acid reflux. In conjunction with consistent physical activity, a healthy and balanced diet can aid in the attainment and maintenance of a healthy body weight.

2. Symptoms of acid reflux during the night can be alleviated by six to eight inches of elevating the head of the bed. While dozing, this angle prevents

gastric acid from flowing back into the esophagus via gravity.

3. Avoid Tight Clothing: Clothing that is too tight around the waist and the girdle can place pressure on the stomach, which may result in acid reflux. Choose apparel with a looser fit to reduce abdominal pressure.

4. Cessation of smoking not only elevates the likelihood of esophageal inflammation but also compromises the integrity of the lower esophageal sphincter, rendering it more susceptible to permit recurrent gastric acid reflux. Cigarette cessation is an essential component of esophagitis management.

5. Implement Stress Reduction Methods: Esophagitis symptoms may be aggravated by stress. By integrating stress reduction techniques into your daily regimen, such as yoga, meditation, or deep breathing, you can enhance your digestive health and overall well-being.

6. Chewing sugar-free gum can increase saliva production, which reduces the risk of reflux and aids in the neutralization of gastric acid.

Avoid varieties containing mint, as it may cause relaxation of the lower esophageal sphincter.

7. Alcohol has the potential to induce relaxation of the lower esophageal sphincter, which in turn can exacerbate acid reflux. Avoid or restrict alcohol consumption, particularly if you are experiencing symptoms of esophagitis.

8. Consistent Physical Activity: Maintain a routine of moderate exercise to promote digestive health as a whole. Physical activity aids in weight maintenance, alleviates tension, and enhances the efficiency of the gastrointestinal system.

9. Meal Timing and Portion Control: It is imperative to exercise mindfulness regarding meal timing and portion measurement. Acid reflux risk can be increased by consuming food near slumber or by consuming substantial meals.

Smaller, more frequent meals may prove to be advantageous.

10. Postprandial Post-Meals: Prevent oneself from falling or reclining immediately following a meal. After a meal, maintain an upright position for a minimum of 45 minutes to facilitate digestion and prevent the reflux of gastric acid into the esophagus.

The concurrent adoption of these lifestyle adjustments and dietary modifications may potentially enhance the efficacy of esophagitis management. It is imperative to seek guidance from healthcare experts, such as dietitians and gastroenterologists, to develop an all-encompassing strategy customized to your particular requirements and guarantee sustained alleviation.

Complete Esophagitis Dietary Guide
Esophagitis, also known as inflammation of the esophagus, presents a formidable management challenge.

Dietary considerations are frequently necessary to mitigate symptoms and promote recovery.

A meticulously planned dietary regimen for esophagitis can substantially aid in the management of the condition. Sample esophagitis diet plans, culinary and preparation advice, monitoring and adjusting the diet, and the significance of consulting a healthcare professional will all be covered in this guide.

Esophagitis Diet Plan Examples
1. Soft foods that are acidic-free:

• Incorporate soft, digestible-friendly foods such as yogurt, liquefied fruits, and oatmeal.

Choose fruits that do not contain acids, such as apples, mangoes, and melons.

Lean proteins such as skinless poultry, fish, and tofu should be selected.

2. Reduced-Fat Options:

• Limit consumption of foods high in fat, as doing so may exacerbate symptoms.

• Make an effort to consume lean cuts of meat, low-fat dairy products, and cooking oils to a minimum.

3. Grains and Vegetables:

By steaming or boiling vegetables, one can achieve a more tender consistency that facilitates digestion.

1. Opt for whole cereals such as quinoa and brown rice, which are rich in fiber and lack an inordinate amount of acidity.

4. Avoid Food Triggers:

• Recognize and abstain from consuming symptom-inducing foods, including citrus fruits, piquant foods, and tomatoes.

• Caffeinc, chocolate, and peppermint should be avoided, as they may irritate the esophagus.

5. Frequent, Small Meals:

One should choose to consume smaller, more frequent meals throughout the day as opposed to three substantial meals.

• A reduced portion size reduces the likelihood of acid reflux and prevents excessive gastric pressure.

6. Sufficient hydration:

• Consistently consume copious amounts of water to support optimal digestion.

• Alcohol, effervescent beverages, and caffeinated beverages should be avoided, as they may worsen symptoms.

CHAPTER FIVE

Advice On Preparation And Cooking

1. Baking and steaming:

One should choose to employ delicate culinary techniques such as steaming and baking to preserve nutrients while preventing the addition of surplus fat.

• Additionally, these techniques soften and enhance the flavor of food for those who have esophagitis.

2. Pureeing and blending:

Consider pureeing or blending vegetables and fruits to make soups and beverages.

• This facilitates the ingestion of a diverse range of nutrients while preventing further irritation.

3. Herbs and Spices as Substitutes:

Herbs such as basil and oregano may be substituted for acidic or peppery seasonings.

One may conduct experiments utilizing mild seasonings to impart flavor without inducing discomfort.

4. Restrictions Regarding Cooking Oils:

Reduce the quantity of cooking oils you use and opt for heart-healthy alternatives such as olive oil.

• Since excessive lipids can exacerbate acid reflux, moderation is essential.

5. Chewing Extensively:

By engaging in comprehensive chewing, one can facilitate optimal digestion and alleviate the strain on the esophagus.

Food particulates that are more minute and thoroughly pulverized are less prone to eliciting irritation.

6. Preventing Overnight Meals:

It is advisable to limit the consumption of substantial meals before slumber to mitigate the potential for acid reflux during the night.

Before lying down, allow a minimum of two to three hours to pass since your last meal.

Observing And Modifying The Diet
1. Maintain a Food Diary:

One should keep a food journal to monitor the correlation between their dietary choices and the manifestation of symptoms.

Make a list of particular foods that elicit distress as well as those that offer solace.

2. Progressive Introductions:

• Gradually incorporate novel foods into the diet to monitor their effects on symptoms.

• By utilizing this method, problematic foods can be identified and a more individualized diet plan can be developed.

3. Caution Regarding Portions:

A portion control system should be implemented to prevent excess, which may be a contributing factor to acid reflux.

• A balanced, smaller diet is more palatable to the digestive system.

4. Observe your body:

• Observe how your body reacts to various substances.

When a specific food item consistently induces discomfort, one should contemplate removing or decreasing its consumption.

5. Periodic Check-ins:

• It is advisable to regularly reevaluate your esophagitis diet in collaboration with your healthcare provider.

• Modifications may be required in response to fluctuations in symptoms or general well-being.

Seeking The Advice Of A Healthcare Professional

1. Auxiliary Nutritional Advice: Consult a registered dietitian or nutritionist for assistance in developing an individualized esophagitis diet plan.

- They have the potential to offer significant insights regarding nutrient needs in the context of symptom management.

2. Medical Assessment:

I strongly advise seeking the expertise of a gastroenterologist or another qualified healthcare professional to obtain a comprehensive assessment of my esophagitis.

In conjunction with dietary modifications, obtain appropriate medical treatment and comprehend the underlying causes.

3. Medication Monitoring:

- When prescribed medications, adhere to the instructions provided by your healthcare provider.

- Certain medications may inhibit the assimilation of nutrients or necessitate modifications in conjunction with dietary modifications.

4. Collaborative Methodology:

Irrespective of the time of day, address both the immediate symptoms and the long-term management of esophagitis in collaboration with your healthcare team.

Consistent follow-up evaluations serve to verify that your dietary regimen maintains its efficacy and remains congruent with your overarching health objectives.

5. Personalized Care:

It is important to acknowledge that esophagitis is a significantly individualized condition, and strategies that prove effective for one individual may not be effective for another.

• With the assistance of your healthcare provider, you can customize a diet plan to your particular requirements and preferences.

In summary, the effective management of esophagitis via dietary interventions necessitates a methodical and individualized strategy.

Consultation with a healthcare professional, adherence to sample esophagitis diet plans, and assistance with cookery and preparation are all essential elements of an effective strategy. Better symptom management and overall health can be attained by individuals with esophagitis through the adoption of informed decision-making and active collaboration with healthcare providers.

Conclusion

Effective management of esophagitis ultimately requires the adoption of a mindful and well-balanced diet. A diet for esophagitis is designed to mitigate symptoms, encourage recovery, and prevent additional inflammation of the esophagus. Avoiding trigger foods and employing dietary practices that alleviate acid reflux are of utmost importance.

A fundamental step is the elimination of acidic, peppery, and fatty foods, as they have the potential to worsen inflammation in the esophagus. Including fruits, vegetables, lean proteins, and whole cereals in one's diet can positively impact digestive health as a whole. It is advisable to consume smaller, more frequent meals to mitigate the risk of reflux and prevent gastric pressure from becoming excessive.

Moreover, adequate hydration is critical for the preservation of a healthy digestive system. Water consumption throughout the day aids in digestion and neutralizes gastric acid. Although dietary modifications are critical, lifestyle modifications such as maintaining a healthy weight, avoiding late-night meals, and avoiding immediately lying down after meals are equally significant.

In the end, it is critical to seek personalized guidance from a healthcare professional or a registered dietitian regarding particular health conditions and triggers that are specific to each individual. Through diligent adherence to a diet that is suitable for individuals with esophagitis, it is possible to effectively manage symptoms and enhance one's overall quality of life.

THE END

www.ingramcontent.com/pod-product-compliance
Lightning Source LLC
Chambersburg PA
CBHW070827290526
45795CB00002B/863